THIS JOURNAL BELONGS TO

TO DO LIST ☑

Notes

INCOMES & EXPENSES

MONTH OF

DATE	INCOME	CATEGORY	AMOUNT
			TOTAL

DATE	EXPENSE	CATEGORY	AMOUNT
			TOTAL

EVERYBODY HAS A DANCING BODY

BRAIN DUMP

GRATITUDE

HOME

WORK

PERSONAL

PROJECTS

OTHERS

NOTES

TO DO LIST ☑

Notes

INCOMES & EXPENSES

MONTH OF

DATE	INCOME	CATEGORY	AMOUNT
			TOTAL

DATE	EXPENSE	CATEGORY	AMOUNT
			TOTAL

WHEN IN DOUBT DANCE IT OUT

BRAIN DUMP

GRATITUDE

HOME

WORK

PERSONAL

PROJECTS

OTHERS

NOTES

TO DO LIST ☑

Notes

INCOMES & EXPENSES

MONTH OF

DATE	INCOME	CATEGORY	AMOUNT
			TOTAL

DATE	EXPENSE	CATEGORY	AMOUNT
			TOTAL

DANCE NOW CRY LATER

BRAIN DUMP

GRATITUDE

HOME

WORK

PERSONAL

PROJECTS

OTHERS

NOTES

TO DO LIST ☑

Notes

INCOMES & EXPENSES

MONTH OF

DATE	INCOME	CATEGORY	AMOUNT
			TOTAL

DATE	EXPENSE	CATEGORY	AMOUNT
			TOTAL

IT IS OKAY TO START OVER

BRAIN DUMP

GRATITUDE

HOME

WORK

PERSONAL

PROJECTS

OTHERS

NOTES

TO DO LIST ☑

Notes

INCOMES & EXPENSES

MONTH OF

DATE	INCOME	CATEGORY	AMOUNT
			TOTAL

DATE	EXPENSE	CATEGORY	AMOUNT
			TOTAL

DO YOU.

BRAIN DUMP

GRATITUDE

HOME

WORK

PERSONAL

PROJECTS

OTHERS

NOTES

TO DO LIST ☑

Notes

INCOMES & EXPENSES

MONTH OF

DATE	INCOME	CATEGORY	AMOUNT
			TOTAL

DATE	EXPENSE	CATEGORY	AMOUNT
			TOTAL

DANCE LIKE THE WORLD IS WATCHING

BRAIN DUMP

GRATITUDE

HOME

WORK

PERSONAL

PROJECTS

OTHERS

NOTES

TO DO LIST ☑

Notes

INCOMES & EXPENSES

MONTH OF

DATE	INCOME	CATEGORY	AMOUNT
			TOTAL

DATE	EXPENSE	CATEGORY	AMOUNT
			TOTAL

THIS IS ONLY THE BEGINNING

BRAIN DUMP

GRATITUDE

HOME

WORK

PERSONAL

PROJECTS

OTHERS

NOTES

TO DO LIST ☑

Notes

INCOMES & EXPENSES

MONTH OF

DATE	INCOME	CATEGORY	AMOUNT
			TOTAL

DATE	EXPENSE	CATEGORY	AMOUNT
			TOTAL

www.ingramcontent.com/pod-product-compliance
Lightning Source LLC
Chambersburg PA
CBHW060406290526
45791CB00002B/632
9781387463695